SHORT BLACKS are gems of recent Australian writing – brisk reads that quicken the pulse and stimulate the mind.

SHORT BLACKS

1 Richard Flanagan *The Australian Disease: On the decline of love and the rise of non-freedom*

2 Karen Hitchcock *Fat City*

3 Noel Pearson *The War of the Worlds*

4 Helen Garner *Regions of Thick-Ribbed Ice*

5 John Birmingham *The Brave Ones: East Timor, 1999*

6 Anna Krien *Booze Territory*

7 David Malouf *The One Day*

8 Simon Leys *Prosper: A voyage at sea*

9 Robert Manne *Cypherpunk Revolutionary: On Julian Assange*

10 Les Murray *Killing the Black Dog*

11 Robyn Davidson *No Fixed Address*

12 Galarrwuy Yunupingu *Tradition, Truth and Tomorrow*

Fat City

Karen Hitchcock

SHORT BLACKS

Published by Black Inc.,
an imprint of Schwartz Publishing Pty Ltd
37–39 Langridge Street
Collingwood VIC 3066 Australia
enquiries@blackincbooks.com
www.blackincbooks.com

First published in the *Monthly*, March 2013.
This edition published 2015.

National Library of Australia Cataloguing-in-Publication entry:
Hitchcock, Karen, author. Fat city / Karen Hitchcock.
9781863957625 (paperback) 9781925203486 (ebook)
Short blacks ; no. 2. Obesity–Australia. Weight gain–Australia.
363.850994

Cover and text design by Peter Long.

FSC www.fsc.org MIX Paper from responsible sources FSC® C009448

Printed in Australia by Griffin Press. The paper this book is printed on is certified against the Forest Stewardship Council® Standards. Griffin Press holds FSC chain of custody certification SGS-COC-005088. FSC promotes environmentally responsible, socially beneficial and economically viable management of the world's forests.

KAREN HITCHCOCK is a doctor and writer. She is the author of an acclaimed Quarterly Essay, *Dear Life*, and an award-winning collection of short stories, *Little White Slips*. She writes a regular column for *The Monthly*.

In the late 1980s I spent a year in the US as an exchange student. The exchange organisation allocated me a local support person named Emily. Emily was white and loud and the fattest person I had ever seen outside a caravan park. She looked different from the rare very fat people I'd seen in Australia. She smelt good and her climate-controlled house meant she did not sweat. She was very well dressed. Her husband was some kind of professional;

I didn't know they even made suits that big.

Emily's family ate like the bejesus. I went to her house once a month for pizza: heavy, oily discs of cheese half a metre across. One each. Before pizza one night I watched the daughter eat a huge bowl of guacamole with a dessertspoon. I couldn't take my eyes off her. I had no concept of calories; I'd simply never seen anyone eat so much avocado in one sitting. I wondered if it would make her vomit. I kept watching as she put down the empty bowl and turned the page of her novel.

I loved Emily. She cared for me the same way she ate: enthusiastically, generously, without restraint. Her bulk did not disgust me. But I never once ate any pizza. The thought of her pizzas made me sick. All those pools of fat. Twenty-five years later I am a physician and Australia is filling up with Emilys.

*

Louise was an educated 35-year-old who had recently lost her high-ranking job and was making ends meet by freelance consulting. Admitted to my ward with pneumonia, she had a high fever and a fast pulse, needed oxygen and was coughing up large amounts of purulent sputum. She was also fat, weighing about 120 kg. I knew that – barring underlying lung disease – obesity was one of the greatest risk factors for life-threatening pneumonia in young people. I felt a responsibility to tell her that her excess fat had harmed her in a way she may not have realised. Every day before my ward round I would say to myself that I was going to broach the subject with her. It seemed a good opportunity to intervene. And yet each time I stood by her bed and looked at her bedside table piled high with literary novels, open blocks of chocolate and teddy-bear biscuits, each time I lifted her pyjama top and pushed my stethoscope into her soft white flesh, I couldn't do it. I was embarrassed to mention her weight; it felt like I was a puritan taking the high moral ground. It felt mean.

As a doctor, I no longer know what to do about the obese. Australians are getting fatter, and our society is geared towards making them that way – consumption doesn't just drive economic growth. So is fatness a doctor's problem? Studies show that verbal interventions during an episode of serious acute illness can result in a change in behaviour – people quit smoking, cut down on their drinking and sometimes lose weight. But usually counselling people to lose weight is hopeless. Then there are the questions of morality, personal responsibility, associated diseases, resource allocation, quality of life and aesthetics. I have moments of clarity – I think of the way Emily ate – and obesity seems simple: more in than out. Then I am engulfed once again by the high science of genetics, by the concept that obesity is a *disease*.

*

I love reading articles with titles like 'How I Lost 25 Kilos', even though the answer is always the same: *I ate less*. Barring the gravely ill and a couple of men, everyone I know wants to lose weight. We live in a society that judges people for being fat, yet has in place every possible means for making them so. Who wants to eat less – of anything – when food is so good and plentiful? It's hard to say no to something that is right in our faces, promising a bit of easy pleasure. It is especially hard to say no when the consequences of overeating come about in such a distant, gradual and mysterious way. I find it difficult to believe that an extra scoop of ice-cream will end up as fat somewhere on my body, even though I know how it happens at the enteric, metabolic and cellular levels. Perhaps this is what happens when we reach the head of the queue and order too much: a fantasy where eating has no consequence, where that pile of French fries and the burger with extra cheese are not our future bodies.

Battles with our appetites and with our bodies are played out on television, in magazines, in the workplace, in families and in hospitals. Be fat in public and you will be weighed by strangers' eyes. The most radical thing on television this past year was the ordinarily flawed 70-kilo naked body of Lena Dunham in *Girls*: little girlish tits above big soft lumps and bumps. How shocking: the protagonist has a paunch and eats cupcakes in the bath. She blatantly displayed her body, a lone counterpoint to the usual stick-insect romantic heroines.

I have heard people say thinness is beautiful and coveted because it is difficult to achieve and rare now, the way curves apparently appeal in times of famine. There are activists who have set out to challenge the fat-is-ugly paradigm, to curb all this body hatred. I am sympathetic to many of their aims. However, their attempts to manipulate what we find beautiful have been crashingly unsuccessful. The Adipositivity Project – which uses artful photographs of morbidly obese half-naked models to reframe fatness as a thing of beauty – remains separatist and marginalised. And the occasional cover shot featuring a so-called plus-sized model is hardly cause for jubilation. These models – often thinner than the nation's average – are freakishly well-proportioned Amazons with flawless faces. The pro-fat bloggers are smart, sassy and pissed off. I'd hang out with them. Yet, if they could click their fingers and be thin, would they? Would Lena Dunham? "I don't want to be skinny like a model," I've had more than one patient tell me, "I'd just like to look like Kate Winslet."

I don't know if there is any force that could purposefully change a culture's definition of beauty. Is fat inherently ugly? Ask Aristotle, Susie Orbach, Naomi Wolf. Their answers are different, their arguments from different places. It is not an empirical question although it reads as one.

Today when we look at those who are thin, part of what we see is a triumph of will over gluttony, so the beauty is a moral beauty; it has little to do with health.

*

Questions of aesthetics aside, obesity is bad because it causes disease by, for instance, raising blood pressure and cholesterol levels, stuffing your liver full of fat, blocking your throat so you can't breathe at night, crushing your joints. Fat people are more likely to get blood clots, gallstones, gout and some cancers – as well as type 2 diabetes, which leads to all manner of medical mayhem. Fat men and women make less money, marry less often and are less educated than the lean. They are more often depressed. In the Framingham Heart Study, which has examined the causes of cardiovascular disease across generations, the very fat lived on average six to seven years less than the lean. The moderately fat lived three years less. If you quit smoking and get fat, you may as well have kept on smoking. These dire facts are not my opinion. They are based on empirical data extracted from large international trials and studies. I wish it were not so. I wish you could get really fat and stay healthy. I wish you could get morbidly obese and be considered beautiful. Maybe it will change with time, as we all become enormous, and we'll look back on the skinny-is-beautiful era with distaste, regarding high cheekbones, defined jaws and long sculptured thighs as skeletal and ugly. I cannot imagine this, but neither could I have imagined that we'd end up in a world so fat.

I listened recently to a neurosurgical registrar describing the difficulty of finding a spinal fracture under 10 centimetres of adipose (fatty) tissue. Neurosurgeons love precision; one false move on the inside and you won't remember your mum. The registrar's voice was filled with a kind of shocked horror. She had to send the car-crash victim to the scanner mid operation, with a metal screw embedded in his neck so the surgeons could find their bearings beneath the mattress of fat. Post-op, none of the neck braces were big enough to fit. To immobilise the man's spine the team used sandbags.

*

This year I started work as the physician in an obesity clinic with a group of bariatric surgeons. No one else really wanted to do it. The attempt to help people lose weight is generally seen as one of the most futile acts we as doctors of internal medicine can perform: pretty much all we can do is make you feel crappier about yourself than you already do. But the surgeons can do something: they can clamp a band at the top of your stomach, cut half your stomach out or bypass part of your small intestine so food is not absorbed. The waiting list for our clinic is long. One of my patients gained 60 kilos between referral and consultation. Some of our patients have become so fat they can walk only five steps without needing a rest. Many are only in their 30s. My role at the clinic is to tighten up their diabetes control, make sure they don't have a catastrophic hormonal condition that has made them fat (no one ever does), treat their high blood pressure and discuss eating and exercise habits. To each patient we show a cartoon of a bolus of food travelling down the surprisingly long oesophagus and squeezing through the junction that leads to the stomach. I watch the food moving down slowly, over and over, one viewing per patient. *This is how your food goes down, so if the surgeons lock a band here, it will take four times as long. You'll have to slow right down when you eat or you will vomit it all back out.*

Now, every time I eat I imagine the food going down my throat, being squeezed by the muscles in my oesophagus before landing with a splat in my smaller-than-I'd-thought stomach. I find myself chewing more and waiting between mouthfuls. Sometimes I even put my fork down on the side of my plate between bites. I'd never done that before; I'd been an eat-and-run kind of girl. I was not at all overweight, but by the third clinic I'd lost 5 kilos.

When my brother was 30, he developed high blood pressure. A general physician checked him out for secondary causes. My brother drank a lot of whisky, smoked, and ate a ridiculous amount of food. It turned out these were the causes. The doctor advised that if my brother religiously took the handful of pills he was about to prescribe, he could get him another 20 years or so. The doctor picked up his pen, opened the script pad. My brother turned white. "Hang on," he said, "I'd like a couple more years than that."

Drugs can help you stay healthy when you are fat, but drugs and doctors cost money. If you are overweight, you cost 25% more per year to keep healthy than a slim person. If you are obese, you cost 45% more. And no drug can fix the functional impairment of being obese. Strap two fully loaded suitcases to the back of someone of normal weight and make them walk up stairs. That only gets them to around 120 kg, which isn't even close to the weight of many patients I see breaking into a sweat on the walk from the waiting room to my office, their knee joints slowly disintegrating. But so what? Motorised scooters are not so expensive. They too could be covered by Medicare.

There are other costs: the fatter you are the greater your ecological footprint. Globally, we are carrying 18.5 million tonnes of excess fat under the skin of the overweight and obese, which – if it were still food rather than adipose tissue – would feed 300 million people for life. Fat people have been compared to petrol-guzzling cars. I feel terrible typing these sentences. I apologise; they are ugly.

*

I met Nora in a diabetes-outpatient clinic. She was 35 years old and had a five-year-old daughter. She had out-of-control diabetes, high blood pressure and fat swelling her liver. She weighed 155 kg and was 150 cm tall, putting her well into the category of morbidly obese. She struggled to lie flat on the examination table; she struggled to rise. Her feet were unkempt, with long yellowed nails and a rim of dark-brown skin cracking around the soles – a disaster waiting to happen for a diabetic, as they are prone to terrible foot infections that sometimes result in amputation. But Nora could not tend to her feet. She could not even see them.

Nora had been listed to have bariatric surgery – in her case, the fitting of a band around the top of her stomach. She said she was terrified of dying during the operation and had cancelled her appointment with the surgeons. I felt sorry for her and wanted to help her. But where to start? I told her that what was going to kill her was her current state of health, not the surgery. I asked her if she wanted to see her daughter grow up and have children. She looked shocked. She started to cry. I told her to go home and empty her cupboards of crap food. Sweet biscuits were her particular weakness. Open the packets, I told her, and dump them. I rebooked her consultation with the surgeons, and gave her the number of a meal-replacement service that she'd had success with in her 20s. Do this for your daughter, I said. She dried her eyes. At the consulting-room door she dropped her handbag and hugged me fiercely. *Thank you, doctor.* But for what? As a registrar in a group clinic, I was unlikely to encounter her again. It is fine to be tough if you are around to temper the consequences for the patient should your intervention fail. What if she couldn't dump the biscuits? What if all I had done was intensify her guilt and self-hatred?

I decided to join the bariatric surgeons because of patients like Nora. In the bariatric surgery clinic I ask my patients for the history of their weight gain, diets they have tried, the state of their health in general, their medication regimens and social situation. It is necessary to get some idea about their eating habits. They sit in the special wide-based chair with their thighs pressed together and hand over food diaries that read like a skinny dietician's. I sit in front of a 280-kilo patient and I keep my tone light and my questions broad: *What do you tend to snack on, when you snack? Is it sweet stuff or salty stuff?* He reads from his diary: *Mid-morning snack: small green apple and two rice crackers.* I continue: *Do you ever feel full? Do you ever keep eating even though you are full? Have you ever eaten to the point of vomiting spontaneously and then kept on eating?* Talking about food is the most difficult and enlightening part of the consultation. The emotion in the room thickens; I am acutely aware of the shame my patients feel. They describe to me what it is like to shop, ride on a bus, take a plane. They tell me that they no longer look into mirrors. I do not ask them to describe the biggest meal they have ever eaten or if they've ever eaten two dozen doughnuts in one sitting. I ask what I need to know to minimise the chances of harming the patients with inappropriate treatments. I do not wish to humiliate them or shame them. I do not wish to turn my fat patients into freaks. It takes time for them to trust me enough to tell me the truth about the mind-boggling volumes of food they consume.

*

I once attended a hospital lecture on the genetic determinants of obesity delivered by a specialist physician. The doctor giving the talk was very fat. As he went on, his face got red and stains of sweat spread from his armpits. Obesity is genetic, he argued, wiping his brow: obesity is a disease. He said: *If you make a fat person thin, you are sentencing them to a lifetime of hunger.*

This depends on your definition of hunger. Eating is not a purely rational, biological act. I can give you a diet that will keep you full all day and make you lose weight, but it won't be very entertaining: it will be mainly made up of watery vegetables like cabbage and celery, egg whites and very lean meat. The pain of abstinence, of unmet desire, is something quite separate from the pain of an empty stomach. The pleasures of eating are complex and multifaceted. In our society, consumption is a form of entertainment and pleasure. Eating is part of this: from the theatre of a meal at a fine-dining establishment to a bag of chips augmenting the television-viewing experience. Most people do not overeat because of a feeling of hunger emanating from the stomach; they are giving in to a desire to consume – they are seeking pleasure or relief, or hoping to fill a void.

I had a friend who had been anorexic and spent her teenage years in and out of hospital, being fed through a nasogastric tube. She recovered in her 20s and managed to channel all of her intrusive obsessional thinking about food into athletics. One day she said to me that she didn't understand why she could be hospitalised against her will for not eating enough, and yet there was no limitation on how fat you could get. It was completely unfair, she said, that you could be refused alcohol if intoxicated but roll into your local fish-and-chip shop 100 kg overweight and be served the equivalent of a week's worth of calories for lunch.

In thousands of labs across the planet, medical researchers are trying to find the cause of, and cure for, obesity. They examine genes, chemical exposures and metabolic pathways. They experiment with amphetamines, anticonvulsants, probiotics. Some of this research is funded by the companies that make and sell the food that makes us fat. In thousands of other labs across the planet, food scientists and marketers are working on ways to make you eat more. They employ highly sophisticated psychological and physiological research to this end; they examine the effects of colour, unit size, price, texture, packaging and advertising on human desire. Look around you: who is winning?

In some ways, scientific research has taken obesity outside the realm where it is a consequence of choices made by a more or less free-willed individual in a more or less free society, which nonetheless disapproves of excess. In current medical research obesity is often conceptualised as an unavoidable disease. It's your genes, your metabolism, the chemicals in your environment, what your mother ate when she was pregnant, whether she fed you at her breast. It is everything but what you choose to put in your mouth.

From a biological point of view, once the stomach has reached capacity, further consumption of food should cause more pain than pleasure. There are well-documented peripheral and central mechanisms – hormones, receptors – that should trigger an aversion to eating any more. But that depends on how strong the pleasure attached to the consumption is. Your stomach is full, but will you say no if I hold my finger dipped in melted dark chocolate to your lips? What if your house is empty and your stomach is full, but you have a bowl full of crunchy somethings sitting in your lap that will make the nothing on television seem bearable? What if inside and out of the house is a constant barrage of powerful images convincing you that the crunchy crap tastes fabulous, and it costs only four dollars for two jumbo packs?

We are attracted to what is forbidden and will resist only if we have a compelling reason to do so: pain, punishment, family disintegration, death. Eating 'bad' food is a relatively benign transgression; you can do it in public, you can do it in the park, in a primary-school playground. The consequences – fatness, disease, early death – are distant enough to be out of sight. Kant famously formulated that no man would sleep with the woman of his dreams if the consequence for him were death immediately afterwards. To stop people consuming vast amounts of the most desirable, calorie-laden, heavily promoted and affordable foodstuffs to appear before our naturally longing eyes, a public-health campaign would need to cause an aversion more powerful than the pleasures promised.

A ban on advertising, graphic counter-campaigns, plain packaging and high taxes have all played a part in making Australia a country with one of the lowest percentages of smokers in the world. How might this approach translate to food? New York City funded an anti–soft drink commercial that showed a man guzzling a glass of blood-streaked liquefied fat. The tagline was "Don't drink yourself fat". Why not plaster packets of chips and chocolate with full-colour photographs of the rot that grows under an apron of fat, or a gangrenous foot caused by diabetes? And if you're thinking, *Eating the occasional chip won't harm me; why punish everyone?*, well, smoking the occasional cigarette won't harm you much either. Any public-health campaign to curb obesity would need to be graphic, to make real the unpleasant consequences of pleasurable excess eating. A drug to treat overeating would need to do the same; not just make people feel full, but render them violently ill if they take an extra bite. But who would take this Kantian drug voluntarily?

*

In the bariatric clinic, we worry most about the compulsive eaters, as well as those who can nominate no other pleasure-seeking activity in their lives besides eating. The question is whether the patient will cope with a life of eating only three saucers of food a day with two little snacks in between. It is dangerous to overeat with a banded stomach. Those who do will vomit profusely, their oesophagus will dilate and may rupture, food can trickle into and infect their lungs. We do not want to cause harm. I explain to the patient: the surgeons are building a door between your body and the food. You have to respect that door; it will only open a crack for a little something to slip in. You must be able to tolerate the limitation.

I ask a young 200-kilo patient what he snacks on. "Nothing," he says. I look him in the eye. *Nothing?* He nods. I ask him about his chronic skin infections, his diabetes. He tears up: "I eat hot chips and fried dim sims and drink three bottles of Coke every afternoon. The truth is I'm addicted to eating. I'm *addicted*." He punches his thigh.

Addicted. The word is useless in my clinic, a mere barrier to any hope of self-determined change. My patient is not addicted; he's a very lonely, unemployed young man who has gradually become socially isolated to the extent that the only thing available to him for comfort and entertainment is food. He has no friends, no money to buy other consumables, little education, no partner, no job. Some days he doesn't leave his bed. The choice for him is to eat this food or experience no pleasure. The surgeon and I discuss his situation, concerned that he may overeat after the band has been fitted. We tell him that surgery may not be appropriate for him, given his situation. The patient is perturbed. "Well, what are you going to do for me if you won't do the operation? Don't you have some kind of ethical responsibility to help me lose weight?"

This is where the obesity-as-disease concept leads us – to a situation in which people demand that medicine shoulder the responsibility. What about the responsibility of the individual? And of society? My patient cries because the highlight of his day is returning from the supermarket with a plastic bag full of junk that he will eat and drink in his empty lounge room. What can I do for him? I can threaten him with his early demise, intensify his shame. I can offer him some evidence-based motivational lifestyle interventions – *swap Coke for Diet Coke!* Prescribe exercise? Walk for an hour at an average pace and you'll only burn off the equivalent of one slice of bread. I could take the old-fashioned approach and wire his jaw shut. I have no hope of resolving his loneliness, his hopelessness, his lack of a job. I could, and do, refer him to a psychologist – if he's lucky he may land one who is talented and sensitive and will try to get to the root of why this young man hates his own guts. More likely he'll be offered a few sessions of behavioural therapy that will make everyone except him feel better.

But he's not like us, is he? He's in the minority; most people are just 20 or so kilos overweight. He's one of those people with an overeating disorder. Actually, I think he is just like most people, but he's got his volume on full. Corporations make it easier for us to eat than to abstain. They loudly promote and supply cheap, taste-intense, non-sating food that is bad for our bodies. They know us better than medicine does. When a fast-food chain dropped its television ads for a weekend, its revenue that week fell by more than 25%. There are more shelves in some supermarkets selling highly processed, nutrient-free combinations of starch, fat, sugar and colouring than there are bearing fresh fruit, vegetables, meat and grains combined. Very few people get obese and none get morbidly obese through the consumption of home-cooked whole foods. To get that fat, for most people, takes piles of highly refined, ready-to-chow junk food and drink. Try googling "what I ate when I was fat".

It is challenging to stay alive at weights above 300 kg. Three hundred is not a threshold – doubtless there is a continuum – but it is the 300 kg–plus people who come to the attention of a hospital, when their bodies start to die around them. I have been involved with, and heard of, a handful of such patients. They were all house-bound because they were no longer able to walk. To remove them from their houses required the state rescue services to demolish door frames. The state's bariatric ambulance must be mobilised. (A standard ambulance can only take a person weighing up to 220 kg.) The patients require special beds, special scanners – sometimes in the zoo – and a small army of medical staff to treat their failing organs. The worst problems involve the skin – it rots and becomes infected when it folds on itself – and the lungs, which are slowly squashed under the mass of flesh so that the patient's intercostal muscles can no longer move to let in the air.

To get that fat takes dedication and persistence. To burn off that much fat is almost impossible. Long-term hospitalisation – a year or more – with a very low calorie diet is really the only path, and even then the person does not leave the hospital in anything like normal shape. The sheets of skin that have grown around the blooming cushions of flesh do not spank back into non-existence. Other consequences of fatness are irreversible. Someone who has never been fat is metabolically healthier (they can eat more) and will live longer than someone who has been fat and no longer is.

A recent *New England Journal of Medicine* article dealing with the rise of chronic lifestyle-driven diseases calls for a change in the way physicians think about their patients. The author suggests that medical students should be taught to be less reductionist, to learn how psychological, social and economic factors all act as determinants of disease. I do not know what medical school is like in the US, but even our surgeons – the most hard-arsed of doctors – sit reeling before the tragic combinations of circumstance and choice that lead our patients to weigh two or three (or four or five) times what they should. The doctors I work with have an excellent grasp of the bio-psycho-social factors that contribute to our patients' states, but we are only doctors. All we have are the tools of our trade: our ears, our voices, our hands, our pills and our scalpels. The waiting rooms are full, the waiting lists are long, the demand is swelling. Obesity is in many ways the logical endpoint of the way we live. Prevention beats palliation, but we'd need psychologists, motivational speakers, social workers, dieticians and physiotherapists to work with us in order to have any hope of tackling the problem. We'd need policy makers and activists. All we have are doctors like me.

Ostensibly cheap food heavily taxes both the individual and the community in terms of disease and redirected health resources. If longevity and the avoidance of disease remain among humanity's aims, we should try to prevent ourselves from getting very fat. Forget obesity as a disease; it's a ruse. For whatever reason, the majority of the population can no longer say *I have had enough*. For whatever reason, the majority of human beings respond to advertisements inviting them to enter a pleasure state by eating a day's worth of calories in one sitting, again and again. In the face of this, we are stuffed. We could say, "You are free agents, totally free, so pay for your own consequences." We could make people pay at the point of choice, via a food tax, or we could limit choice. The other option, always unspoken, is: let us have our cake. Let's just eat and eat, get fatter and fatter, and work out how best to live with it. This is where we are heading now: fatness, outside of morality, as an accepted consequence of the world as we have made it.

We can decide as a country, as a world, that we are going to consume what we have until we're done, eating as much as we wish and treating all the concomitant diseases by diverting substantial amounts of government revenue into medicine and pharmaceuticals. If we do choose this path – and we are most of the way there already – we must be honest about what we are choosing to do: to spend our country's money on the consequences of indiscriminate consumption.

If you come to me, your doctor, and you ask me to make you thin, for now I will have to cut you or drug you, as these are the only weapons I have to ward off the sirens. There will come a time when patients stop asking their doctors to make them thin. It will either be because fatness is rare again, or because it has become entirely accepted. The choice is in your hands. Are you going to eat it?

SHORT BLACKS

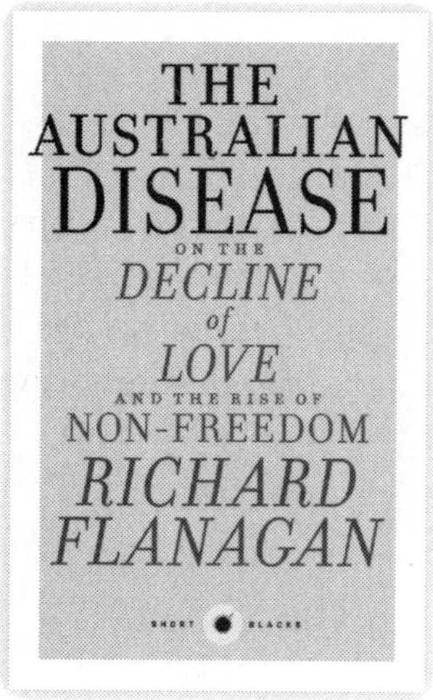

Richard Flanagan's perceptive, hilarious, searing exposé of the conformity that afflicts our public life.

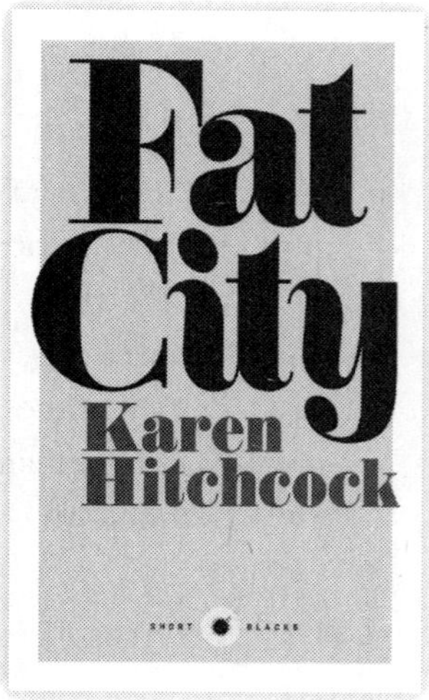

In a riveting blend of story and analysis, doctor and writer Karen Hitchcock explores chemistry, psychology and impulse to excess to explain the West's growing obesity epidemic.

WWW.SHORTBLACKS.COM

CLASSIC SHOTS OF AUSTRALIAN WRITING

Robyn Davidson's fascinating and moving essay about nomads explores why, in times of environmental peril, the nomadic way with nature still offers valuable lessons.

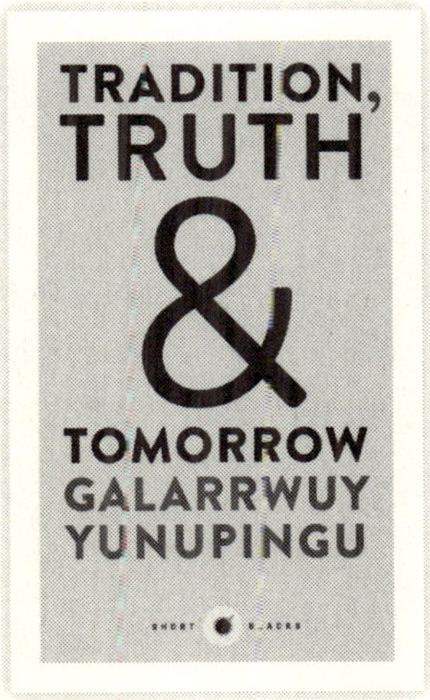

Galarrwuy Yunupingu tells of his early life, his dealings with prime minsters, and how he learnt that nothing is ever what it seems.